SURVIVE COVID

SURVIVE COVID BY STAYING ALKALINE

Dr Eapen Koshy

Foreword by
Prof. K.N. Vasupalaiah & Dr Rathna Vasupal
Founder & 1st Crown Ambassador Couple, DXN INDIA

Konark Publishers Pvt Ltd
New Delhi • Seattle

Konark Publishers Pvt Ltd
206, First Floor,
Peacock Lane, Shahpur Jat,
New Delhi - 110 049
Tel : +91-11-4105 5065
e-mail : india@konarkpublishers.com
website : www.konarkpublishers.com

Konark Publishers International
8615, 13th Ave SW,
Seattle, WA 98106
Phone : (415) 409-9988
e-mail : us@konarkpublishers.com

Copyright © Dr Eapen Koshy, 2021

All rights reserved. No part of this book may be reproduced or utilised in any form or by any means, electronic or mechanical, including photocopying, recording, or by any information storage and retrieval system, without prior permission in writing from the publisher. The views and opinions expressed in this book are the author's own and the facts are as reported by him, which have been verified to the extent possible, and the publisher is not in any way liable for the same.

Disclaimer: This book is intended only for reference, and is not a medical manual. The information given by the author is designed to help you make informed decisions about your health. It is not intended to replace medical advice for any treatment prescribed by your doctor.

ISBN: 978-81-949286-4-5
Editors: Ranjana Narayan & Preeta Priyamvada
Cover jacket: Misha Oberoi
Icons@Shutterstock
Printed and bound at Thomson Press (India) Ltd

*Dedicated to
Mother Earth*

Truth stands, even if there be no public support. It is self-sustained.
—Mahatma Gandhi

Contents

Foreword	*viii*
Advance Praise	*xi*
A Word from the Publisher	*xiii*
Introduction	*xv*
1. What is Alkalinity?	1
2. How Alkaline are You?	4
3. Innate and Adaptive Immunity	14
4. Ladder of Alkalinity	22
5. Beating the Cytokine Storm in Covid	30
6. Alkaline Superfoods	41
7. The Post-Covid Body Status	54
8. The Planetary Interconnection	60
9. Earth Synchronicity, Earth Humility	65
10. The Developed World and Alkalinity	70
11. Will Humans Become Extinct? Quite Possibly	75
12. The Way Forward	83
Conclusion	*85*
Common Questions	*88*
Reference List	*95*
A Promise	*102*

Foreword

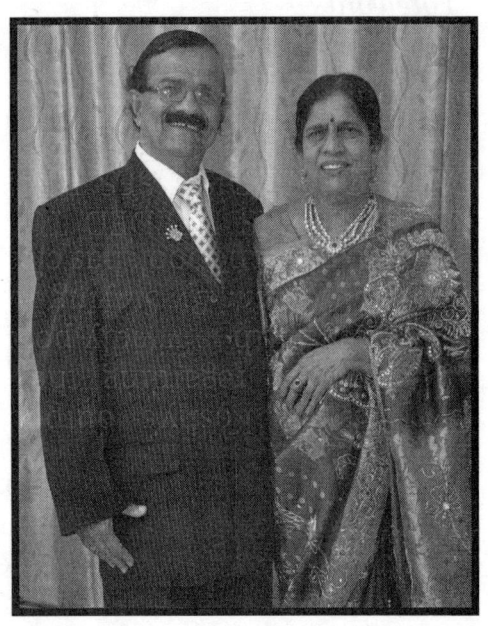

Prof. K.N. Vasupalaiah,
MA, MPhil (Economics)
Dr Rathna Vasupal,
MBBS, FCGP, FCIP, FAGE, ECFMG (USA)
Founder & 1st Crown Ambassador Couple, DXN INDIA

Foreword

Dr Eapen Koshy's outpouring of pent-up emotions regarding the unceasing abuse of Mother Earth is vividly portrayed in his book *Surviving Covid: By Staying Alkaline.* Dr Koshy, through this handbook has clearly depicted WHY ALKALINITY IS NEEDED TO END THE ROOT CAUSE OF ALL DISEASES. This is an extraordinary investigation by a super specialist modern plastic surgeon.

This incredible book is a result of Dr Koshy's experience from using Mother Nature's gifts to mankind on himself and his patients through his clinical practice for over 40 years. He is of the firm opinion that lifestyle diseases will only come to an end if we make modifications to our food habits. He concludes that we just see the tip of the iceberg of modern pandemics. If we do not take action on a war footing then there is a fear that the human race will go extinct. He truthfully states that we are responsible for this disaster, deservingly, for not respecting Mother Earth. His vexation is felt quite strongly over the lingering unacceptance of many people that Mother Nature's gifts are paramount to healing humanity.

Many natural healing techniques using plants and herbs are beyond modern medicine and scientific evidence. However, recent breakthroughs in clinical trials on nutrition around the globe on human health and evidence of superior herbs like Spirulina and Ganoderma are now well documented by allopaths, who have evinced interest in using these herbs as adjuvants or as alternative treatment. The world has woken up to immunomodulating natural herbs during this pandemic. The final Q&A section perspicuously explains everything for any layman to understand.

In the end, this book of uncommon sense and unconventional wisdom is a must for all who are concerned about health, prevention from diseases, nature and humanity. We wholeheartedly thank Dr Koshy for yet another indispensable tool for the benefit of humanity and all those who are concerned about wellness through prevention.

Chennai,
15 June 2021

Advance Praise

There are few allopathic medical doctors who understand the roots of illness and the pillars of wellness. Dr Eapen Koshy clearly understands this and has helped millions to further this knowledge. Practically, he has demonstrated this via his medical and surgical outcomes. It is purely amazing and true. In this book, he simplifies the concept of alkalinity for anyone to appreciate and grasp. It is applied to our daily choices, thus unequivocally empowering the reader. Dr Koshy is a mentor, teacher and authority on wellness.

Dr Patrick Ijewere, *B.Pharm, MD (Howard University USA), Int. Medicine (John Hopkins USA), MBA*
Medical Director
The Nutrition Hospital & Wellness Center, Ikoyi, Lagos, Nigeria

A Word from the Publisher

Dear Readers,

The world is presently grappling with a catastrophe of gigantic proportions. The Covid-19 pandemic has stopped the world in its tracks. With millions affected across the globe, and hundreds of thousands dead and dying, any ray of hope in the form of an answer to fight the pandemic is what people are seeking.

Dr Eapen Koshy, who belongs to India and is

practising in Nigeria at present, is a votary of an alkaline way of life—in which respect for Mother Nature is foremost—to increase the body's immunity to fight, not just the Covid-19 virus but all illnesses, and stay healthy and fit.

We hope this book, brought out in quick time by Konark, proves useful to readers, and offers some hope.

25 April 2021 **K.P.R. Nair**
New Delhi

Introduction

We are in the midst of a pandemic. A single virus, the Covid-19, has caused over two million deaths on our planet, during 2020 and 2021. However, it is not the virus to blame. It is our own weakened immune systems that have responded with fatal inflammatory responses. Acidic food intake, electromagnetic radiation pools and an immune-lowering lifestyle has led to the weakening of our immune systems. We have unwittingly become the prisoners of our own war; a war that is lowering our immune systems to such an extent that a mass extinction may be a possibility.

Only a strong immune system can save us. The answers to the current pandemic and to future pandemics lie in alkalinizing our body to boost our immune system and maintain this with an immune-friendly lifestyle. We need a higher shift in our thinking, and need to move to simpler earth-synchronous ways of life. This alone can take our planet to an age with no pandemics, and to an age with no violence or intolerance, as an alkaline body will nurture a calm, inclusive and tolerant alkaline mind.

To understand this fully, we need to unlearn a lot and be humble. This book explains, in a simple manner, how such a state can be achieved. I truly wish you all a full understanding.

Dr Eapen Koshy

The answers to immunity
Must be man-made
That is what I thought
I burned the midnight oil
Studied very many books
But now I know
The answers I was searching for
Were around me all the while
Mother Earth has all the answers
Saved for us, in her treasure trove.

Eapen Koshy

1
What is Alkalinity?

Life on earth depends on an appropriate pH level within and around us. This is true for all living beings, whether on land or in the sea.

Our body is a wonderful creation of trillions of dynamic cells—varying in density and size—all interrelated and communicating with each other and working in harmony. For an optimal function of every body cell, the pH balance has to be at 7.4 or close to it. The pH of 7 is neutral, 0 is most acidic and 14 is most alkaline. For sustainable life, the pH level must be at 7.4 or close to it.

The body pH status is the resultant manifestation of all ongoing metabolic and detoxifying processes in the body. The pH balance determines our health status more than any other parameter. The white blood cells, which are on the frontline of our immune system and protect us from illnesses, become lethargic and weakened in an acidic pH balance; and they get immediately perked up and are alert when a body has an alkaline pH balance.

In the modern era, when lifestyles are stress-ridden and there is ignorance about, or not enough attention to, healthy food habits, there is an acidic overload in our bodies. This results in a constant challenge for our bodies to maintain the alkaline pH of 7.4.

A person is in an *alkaline balance* if all cells and organs are *at ease* in maintaining this pH of life. A person is in an *acidic balance* if all cells and organs are *working overtime* and are at a breakdown threshold trying to maintain this pH of life.

A well-oxygenated alkaline balanced body has adequate immunity to successfully fight diseases. Diseases occur in a body that has low-oxygenated, acidic cells as its immunity becomes weak. This happens because of nutrient-deficient toxic diet, toxic emotions and a toxic lifestyle.

The current pandemic experience has hit us really hard, and it has now become urgent that every citizen of the world is aware of ways to boost immunity and practice a healthy, immunity-friendly lifestyle. It is important to learn to maintain an alkaline body and follow an alkaline diet. Every school curriculum should have this subject incorporated.

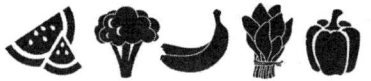

2

How Alkaline are You?

*Let food be thy medicine, and
let medicine be thy food.*
—**Hippocrates**

Hippocrates (410–360 BC) is considered the 'Father of Modern Medicine' and was regarded as the greatest physician of his time. He practiced medicine in Greece, and travelled to Egypt and Libya as well and practiced there too. His medical acumen and approach to disease were far beyond his times. Historical records show he recommended diet and exercise for all ailments and medicinal plants for some ailments. He stressed on seeing the body as a whole and not in parts. Unfortunately, we have moved away from his teachings in the present times. In the current times of specialists and chemical drugs, we have, in many ways, lost our way.

We are What We Eat

Nutrients derived from our food determine the structure, foundation and energy levels of all our cells and our immune systems. All food items that we consume are either acid-producing or alkaline or neutral. Thus, by being aware of the nature of the food that we eat, and by taking care of our diet and choosing wisely what to eat, we can maintain our body's pH balance and improve our immunity. However, this cannot happen with one meal or an occasional healthy diet. It can be achieved only by adopting proper diet as a regular way of life.

Unfortunately, modern-day medical practitioners and even nutritionists do not have a true understanding of alkaline nutrition or its

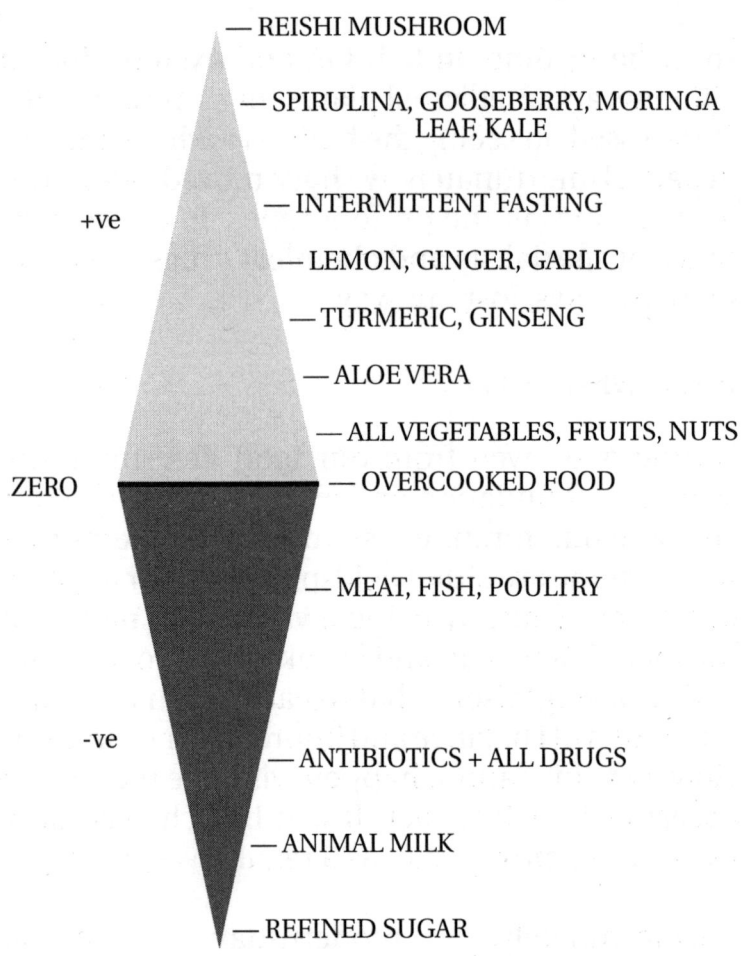

Fig 2.1: Immunity Nutrition

importance. A real doctor is one who understands nutrition.

Figure 2.1 shows two pyramids. The pyramid on the top shows alkaline nutrition, and the pyramid below shows acidic nutrition. The central line depicts neutral nutrition.

Some Foods With Acidifying Effect

Refined white sugar is the most acidifying food that people consume almost daily. Regular sugar intake is akin to a slow suicide. A slow and steady loss of physical and mental equanimity follows as the body gradually acidifies. The world is on a sugar overload now; to counter its effect, people need to add something bitter to their lives.

A bottle of coke has a pH value of 2.5, with around 10 teaspoons or more equivalent of refined sugar. To neutralize the acidic pH produced by one bottle of coke, our body requires 32 glasses of alkaline water with a pH of 10. Calcium from our large reservoir base in our bones and muscles are released into our blood circulation for pH homeostasis, with our kidneys working overtime. It is estimated that half our skeletal mass can be excreted in our urine over 20 years to balance our sugar diet acid overload. To prevent an osteoporotic skeletal mass 20 years from now, sugar intake should be stopped without any further delay. It follows that our skeletal mass and strength can be maintained by consuming an alkaline diet.

Animal milk and milk products are also acid producing, mucus producing, and cardiac unfriendly. A cow weans off its calf by the time it is six months old. It makes no sense for us to be drinking its milk all our life, with growth hormones and concentrated fat and other hormones meant for a neonate calf. Ice cream and milk byproducts like cheese are concentrated forms of milk and compete with sugar for the most acidifying of all foods in current age.

Similarly, meat and animal products also fall in this category. Red meat and processed meat, common in modern-day diet, are acid-producing foods. Over and above the high protein content, the phosphorous in all meat products contribute to the acidic load. Eggs further add to the acidic load. The post-meal tiredness is in fact the result of the kidneys and all cells of the body trying to cope with acidity.

An acidic balance weakens the white blood cells and makes them unable to combat disease and downgrades immunity. It decreases energy production within the cell mitochondria, causes tumor cells to form and thrive, and promotes fatigue and illness. A blood pH of 7 or below will cause coma, gasping, and death.

The root cause of all lifestyle diseases is the underlying acidic body balance. No one with an alkaline body balance would succumb to the Covid-19 virus as in an alkaline body there is no inflammatory hyper response, and innate and adaptive immunity would be working smoothly. Alkalinity does not follow a rule book. It is a continuous journey; it is a way of life. One has to conquer each day with alkalinity and keep going up the alkaline ladder.

Neutral Food

Overcooked food is devoid of any nutritious capacity and does not give any positive nutrition to the body.

Alkaline Nutrition

All of earth's produce is alkaline. All vegetables and fruits and all soil produce are alkaline. That is, they result in alkalization of the body. In addition, these earth products provide antioxidant effect, adaptogen effect, positivity, and pure energy. They are nature's alkaline pharmacy.

Some foods of daily intake are not very acidic outside the body but leave large acidic residue when processed in the body. Animal milk is a classic example. Some foods are acidic outside but become alkaline once ingested. Lemon and tomatoes are examples of these; high antioxidant content and specific enzymes make them alkaline. In Figure 2.1, ginger, lemon, turmeric, aloe vera, ginseng root, etc. are foods that have more alkalinity and antioxidants packed in them. They could be called tonics. It is the alkalinity that gives the tonic effect. Turmeric, further, has a large content of zinc which is needed in all steps of the immune antibody response.

Foods that have alkalinity and have nutrients densely packed within them are gooseberry, moringa leaves, avocado, berries, leafy greens, quinoa, olives, and nuts, among others. Spirulina, a blue green alga, and some varieties in the mushroom family top the list of superfoods that have maximum alkalinity. Due to soil depletion and overzealous use of pesticides and chemical fertilizers, most vegetables have lost their inherent nutrient power. The cauliflower we eat today does not have the nutrient content of the cauliflower our grandparents had. In view of the decrease in the nutritional value of the vegetables that we have today, these superfoods should be included in our diets now.

A practice that helps to make the body alkaline is fasting. It induces alkalinity as the body goes into a detoxifying mode—insulin production tapers down, and glucagon, growth hormone, adrenal hormones, and the like are released and the body goes into a hormonal celebration. Hence, fasting has a prominent position on the alkaline nutrition chart.

The commonest symptoms of acidic overload are acne, menstrual cramps, feeling of sighing, water retention, insomnia, hyperirritability, easy to anger, selfish outlooks, inability to hold breath for 20 seconds, etc. A body with high acidic food intake will be lethargic, will fall sick frequently with repeated urinary infections, will have frequent headaches, and will have bad mouth and body odor. As acidic balance rises, the body invites cancer, hypertension, diabetes, and renal failure. An acidic body will harbor an acidic mind, which is a mind in pre anger, filled with suspicions, selfishness, feelings of superiority, forgetting earth synchronicity, and nurturing a false ego and pride. An acidic mind is incapable of listening to what Mother Earth is telling us.

Alkaline foods prevent the leeching of calcium from the bones. They thus help in maintaining bone health for years to come, help fight free radical damage, reduce inflammation, and support cell regeneration so that the body can thrive.

An alkaline body is disease-free, with no lifestyle diseases. No cancerous changes can occur in an alkaline body. Alkalinity enables the body to follow the circadian rhythm of life. It also nurtures an alkaline mind which is a calm, all-inclusive mind, capable of listening to Mother Earth, and appreciates her magnificence.

Think for yourself now. How alkaline are you?

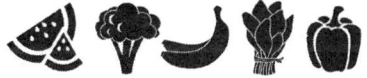

3

Innate and Adaptive Immunity

A fortress is where kings and ministers took refuge. It was a place where the enemies could not penetrate. Depicted in Figure 3.1 is a 400-year-old fortress in Vellore, in South India. The major modes of its defence are the thick walls constructed with solid rocks and the water body surrounding the fort. If the enemy succeeded (which happened rarely) in crossing the barrier and getting inside, then the second line of defence

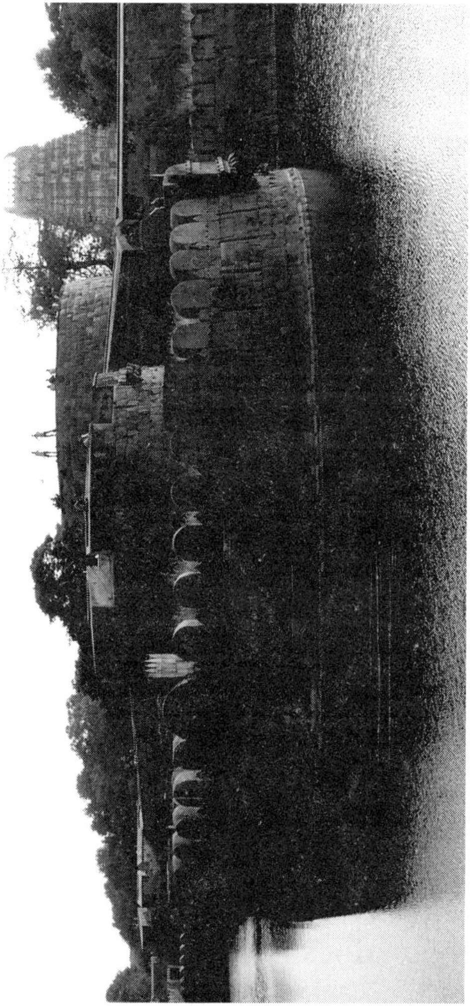

Innate and Adaptive Immunity

Fig 3.1: Vellore Fort built in the 16th century

would be the king's army, ready to neutralize each enemy individually.

Our body's immune defence is very similar. We have an innate defence which is a non-specific defence against all pathogens (first line of defence). We also have adaptive or antibody response (second line of defence) which is specific to the pathogen and has a memory of its own. Just as the walls of a fort can age and become fragile, the body's innate defence mechanisms also weaken with age. But as the king's army is reinforced inside the fort with more young men as the need arises so that the defence remains young and strong, similarly, the adaptive immunity of our body keeps making fresh antibodies all the time so that our immunity does not weaken with age.

A fascinating phenomenon of the body is that a man in his eighth decade can still produce sperms which are capable of fertilizing an ovum and producing a normal child. Similarly, the antibody production does not reduce in quality with age.

The innate immune system is non-specific and does not allow any pathogen to enter the body. They are physical, chemical, or biological barriers. Innate immunity alone is enough to ward off a majority of pathogens that may enter our body. Our skin, all epithelial surfaces, cilia in the respiratory tract, acidic gastric juice, phagocytes, our own commensal flora of bacteria and viruses, our body pH and cellular pH are all part of our innate immunity.

Fever, inflammatory circulatory response, phagocytes that enlarge themselves and line the alveoli in the lungs and gastrointestinal tract, and mucosal lining are all a part of our innate immunity defence. The innate immune defence holds no memory. Just like the walls of the fortress, they are just there and are sufficient against a majority of the pathogens.

Adaptive immunity

To understand this, let us now encounter the king's army inside the fort. The adaptive immune system must be a result of the evolutionary process from and beyond the innate immune system as only the vertebrates have the adaptive immune system.

To describe in a basic way, T lymphocytes and B lymphocytes develop from progenitor cells in the bone marrow. The B cells remain in the bone marrow during the development while the T cells migrate in the circulation and develop in the thymus gland; hence their names. Both are capable of identifying and starting processes of neutralizing foreign antigens. They are also capable of recognizing one's own antigens or auto antigens.

An antibody (formerly known as an immunoglobulin) is a large Y-shaped protein produced by B-cells to identify and neutralize foreign objects such as bacteria and viruses. Though the general structure of antibodies is similar, a small region at the tip of the Y structure is extremely variable, allowing millions of antibodies with different antigen binding sites to exist. This region is known as the hypervariable region.

Thus, the hypervariable portion is able to form a binding site to neutralize any new antigen that is encountered. The base of the Y plays a role in modulating the immune cell activity, especially facilitating phagocytosis.

It is a truth that had people not experienced the distress caused by the Covid pandemic, nobody would read these lines with interest. The fact is that there is no life possible without a working immune system. When all is going well, we do not want to know anything about it.

The 1984 Nobel prize in physiology or medicine was awarded jointly to Niels K. Jerne, Georges J.F. Köhler, and César Milstein. These three could be called the 'Fathers of Modern Cellular Immunology'.

Jerne, a theoretician, noted that once an antigen is encountered and the antibody is created to neutralize it, then that antibody cell has the preferential property conferred on it to proliferate when needed. Thus, a Darwinian natural selection of antibody preference occurs here amongst billions of antibodies in the immune system.

Köhler and Milstein developed the hybridoma technology to produce monoclonal antibodies. Their work was fascinating and has a huge potential to change many therapies for cancer and infections. They succeeded in fusing an antibody cell and a myeloma (plasma cancer cell), thus producing an antibody clone production which has the speed to replicate at the same rate as a cancer cell, a property they get from the myeloma parent cell.

However, practically this encountered much side effects. The huge antigen antibody complexes formed could not be cleared by the spleen and liver, and this gave rise to arterial and venous blood clots, hepatitis, and cerebrovascular events.

In fact, we are seeing these coagulation events in many Covid patients in their later stages and also after vaccination. This is because the immune system is not healthy enough in these individuals to remove the antigen antibody complexes with ease. In a healthy alkaline body, these are removed

Innate and Adaptive Immunity

immediately from the circulation by the spleen, liver, and kidneys.

Just as all body cells are in constant communication with each other in a healthy body, the immune cells and lymphokines are dependent and in communication mostly with the neurological and endocrine systems. Therefore, positivity and a happy mind is most important to maintain healthy immunity.

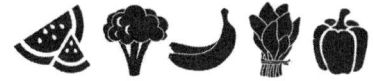

4

Ladder of Alkalinity

*You have the freedom to be yourself,
your true self, here and now,
and nothing can stand in your way.*
   —**Richard Bach** in his book
Jonathan Livingston Seagull

Alkaline Ladder

As the body becomes alkaline, one becomes earth synchronous and one's body and mind become more in line with the unchanging universal

Ladder of Alkalinity

> JONATHAN is an ordinary seagull bored and frustrated with materialism, conformity, and limitations of everyday seagull life. He starts experimenting with flights, does daring aerial feats, and finds himself transcending to a higher form. He finds others like him and he understands that a seagull is an unlimited idea of freedom. To go up the ladder he learns that 'love for everything' and 'ultimate forgiveness' are mandatory conditions he has to pass along the way up.

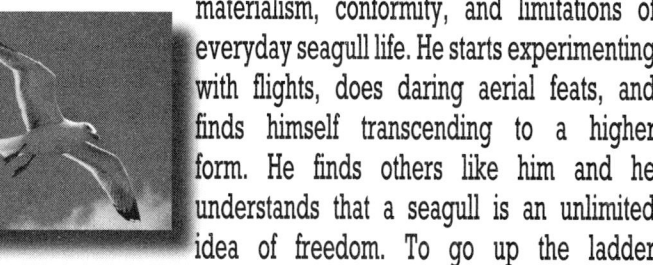

laws. The alkaline ladder does not mean deeper into the alkaline pH, but it implies *spending more living time in alkalinity*. Similarly, for acidic pH balance, I remind the reader that life needs the maintenance of a pH within a small range.

Figure 4.1 depicts the alkaline–acidic chart and the attributes at various levels of acidic and alkaline balances. The circle is my impression of the world population status now. The bottom red portion of the chart is acidic balanced bodies. These are populations with lifestyle diseases and chemically controlled blood pressures, blood

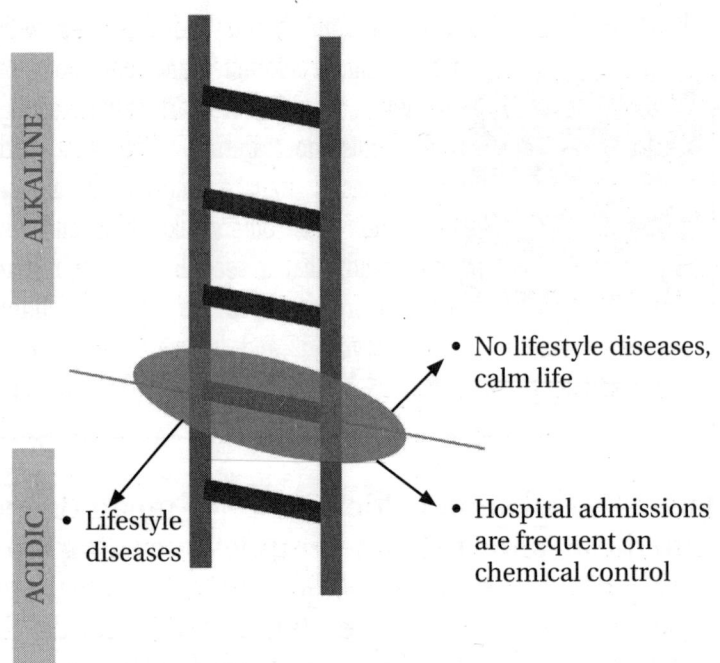

Circle depicts world status now

Fig. 4.1: Alkaline–Acidic Chart

sugars, cholesterol levels, etc. The chemical drugs ensure that they can never come out of the acidic state as all chemicals further acidify our cells.

Ladder of Alkalinity 25

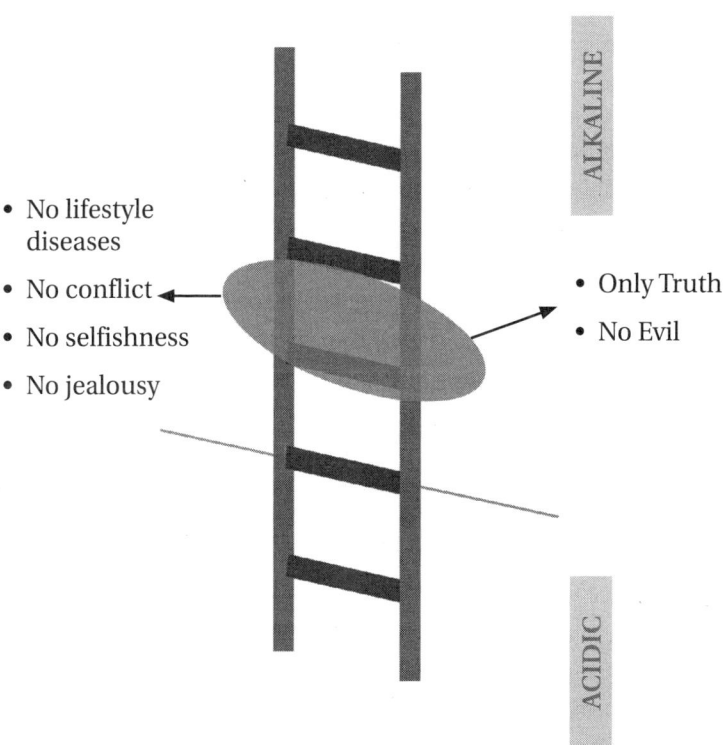

Fig. 4.2: Next Phase of Alkalinity

Acidic bodies will also harbor acidic minds characterized by selfishness, easy to anger, feelings of superiority, feelings of exclusivity, and their lifestyles will not be earth synchronous.

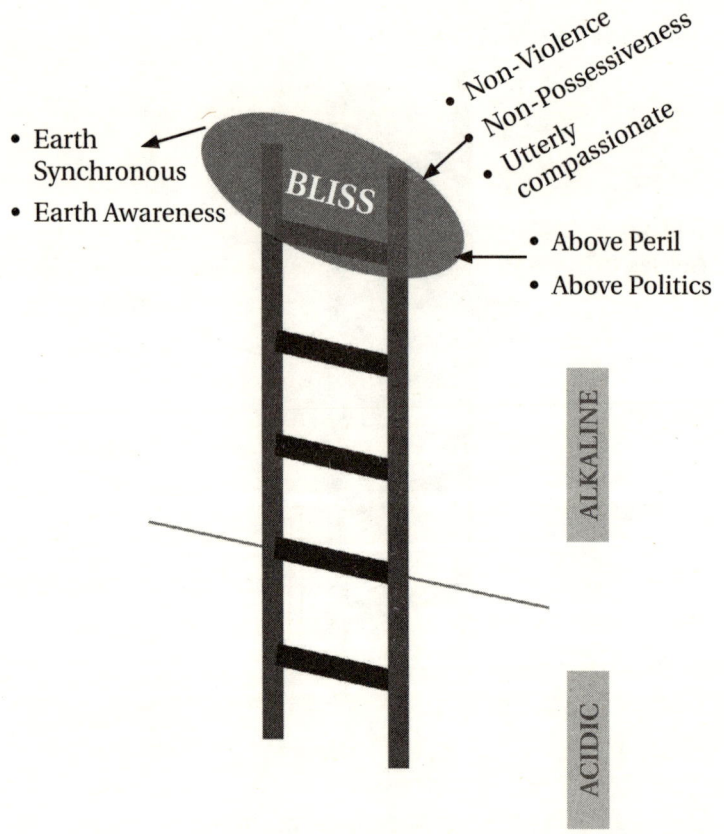

Fig. 4.3: Pinnacle of Alkalinity

They cannot appreciate the magnificence of the earth and cannot relate to even fellow beings, let alone animals and plants. They would be bogged down by religious, race, and regional exclusivities.

The upper half of the circle will be individuals and societies in an alkaline balance. They will not be hospital birds and will have a broader outlook to life and surroundings. They would not fall sick often and will make an attempt to stop polluting the environment. I believe that 50 per cent of the current world population would be here.

If the entire population was in this circle of alkalinity, there would be no hospitals needed to cure diseases. Doctors would only be treating trauma. In such a scenario, the doctors will understand alkalinity and practice preventive medicine. For example, the physician would be telling an elderly patient that he is predicting a cardiac event in a year's time unless the patient changes his/her nutrition and adds more exercise in their routine. How much better this would be rather than performing an angioplasty on a patient after a heart attack. If the patient has a heart attack, then his physician has failed him.

Within this circle, countries would not have border patrols, and there would be no wars. In such a state, people would realize the futility of war. Ego, insecurities, lust of power, desire to control others, anger, and bitterness kind of emotions would not exist anymore. Religious, ethnic and such differences would be tolerated with more grace, and truth alone would matter, be followed, and respected. In this kind of a scenario, there also would be no sickness and there would be no need for hospitals or prisons.

The circle on the top depicts the pinnacle of alkalinity. Total earth synchronicity and earth humility exists at this stage. One would realize that there is only truth and goodness around us. Evil does not exist outside us. It can only exist within us and comes from within us. One would thus have no evil mindset. Once evil ceases to exist, truth is not needed any more. At this state, religions would not be needed. One would rise above truth and religions. One would be in a state of bliss and in complete synchronicity with earth, and be able to relate to all of earth's living beings and plants. People would be as much concerned about animal rights as about human rights. Animals would be loved, nurtured, taken care of, and allowed to live freely.

In such a state, death will not be from sickness, as no sickness can occur in such a state. Death will be by choice, when one would tell Mother Earth that one has seen and enjoyed enough and now wishes to return to her. In fact, one would yearn to go back to soil and welcome death.

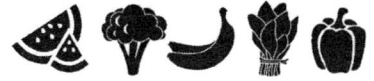

5

Beating the Cytokine Storm in Covid

Prevention is the Cure

Cytokine storm (severe immune response) occurs in Covid infections commonly by the eighth day once innate immunity has failed and one progresses from non-pulmonary stage to pulmonary inflammation stage. The viral load is now high and the lungs are in a state of inflammation. All inflammatory markers will be high and CT scans of the lungs will show the typical ground glass appearances (opacities or hazy gray areas) of varying degrees. In an alkaline, immune-competent body, this storm would not occur.

Turmeric – Nature's Gift

Turmeric is the ultimate answer to prevent and treat cytokine storm. Drink one glass of warm water with one full teaspoon of turmeric powder stirred into it. Repeat again after one hour. The hypoxia (low oxygen in tissues) and distress will start settling.

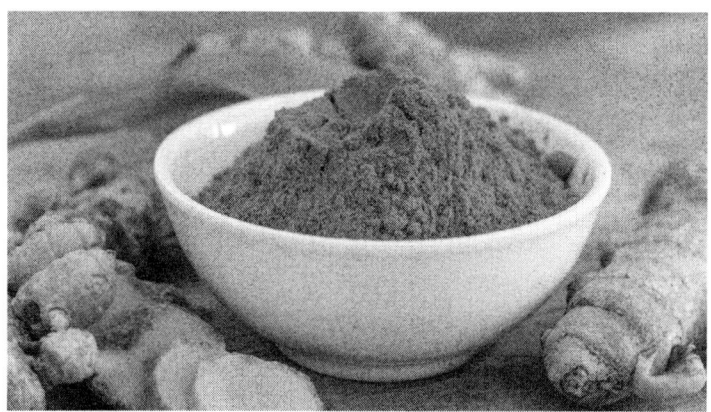

Image Courtesy: freepik.com

Turmeric is highly alkaline and contains the chemical 'curcumin' which has profound anti-inflammatory, antioxidant and anti-viral properties. No chemical drugs are available that can upgrade immunity and counter the cytokine response. Curcumin (turmeric) can and should be used as a therapeutic agent and results in suppressing the cytokine response and hypoxia. There are innumerable papers and plenty of animal studies providing compelling evidence of its therapeutic use in viral pneumonias. People who consume turmeric daily by mixing turmeric powder in lukewarm water are highly protected against developing a cytokine storm response. Various preclinical studies have found that intranasal administration of curcumin into lungs relieved inflammation. One can, thus, add turmeric powder to water in steam inhalation.

During the ongoing Covid-19 pandemic, everyone should be using this 'queen of spices' from the kitchen cabinet. The breathlessness settles in one hour after taking warm water infused with turmeric.

If taken daily, turmeric powder in warm water is the best prevention and gives the body the daily upgrade in alkalinity. There are at least four cytokine pathways that curcumin regulates and modulates. The more inquisitive reader can look up the many published medical journals on this (Lodha R. et al. 2000; Ziteng Liu, et al. 2020).

In younger individuals, the cytokine response may be due to a strong immune system and even here curcumin modulates the cytokine response and prevents it.

Ginger

Ginger has profound anti-inflammatory, anti-cancer and antioxidant properties. It is always best to use fresh ginger—either with the peel intact or chewed raw—for maximal effects.

Ginger has a different line of action from curcumin in its anti-inflammatory mode of action. It behaves as Cyclooxygenase-2 (COX-2) inhibitors (a type of nonsteroidal anti-

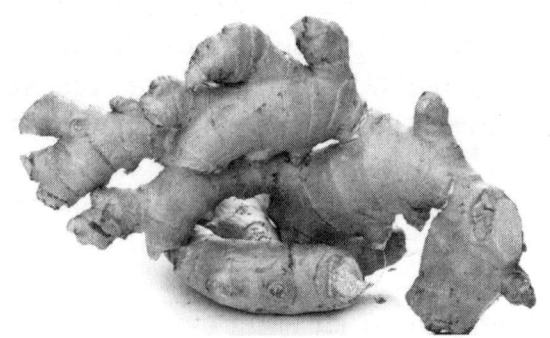

Image Courtesy: freepik.com

inflammatory drug) do and is an ideal adjuvant to curcumin (Srivastava K.C. et al 1992; Frondoza C.G. et al 2004.)

Together, ginger and turmeric boast some synergistic health benefits. If a small piece of ginger is chewed alongside drinking the turmeric water, the anti-inflammatory property of curcumin is augmented and recovery from hypoxia is speeded up.

Garlic

Garlic has strong anti-viral and moderate anti-inflammatory properties. It is best when swallowed raw on an empty stomach.

If a small garlic pod is swallowed along with turmeric powder water and a small piece of ginger, then the resultant anti-inflammatory and antioxidant actions are like the unleashing of raw earth power and the cytokine storm gets averted.

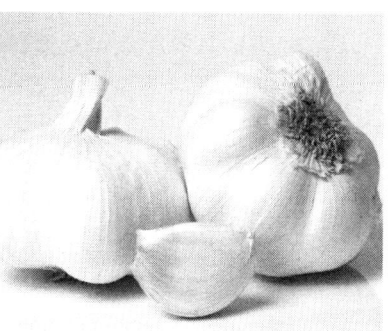

Image Courtesy: freepik.com

Lemon

One should make it a habit of chewing and swallowing a small piece of lemon along with the peel. Lemon peel that we usually discard contains five to ten times more vitamins than the lemon juice.

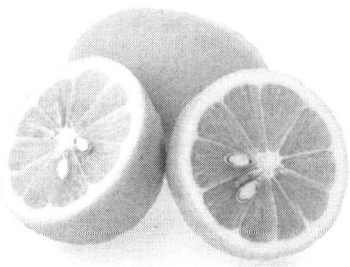

Image Courtesy: freepik.com

Though lemon is acidic, it is packed with antioxidants and has a very alkalizing effect on the body. It further augments the antioxidant properties of all the above herbs and spices. Lemon is a known powerhouse of vitamin C—a key nutrient for supporting one's immune system. The vitamin C gives a wake-up boost and helps in hydration of cells.

When the body's innate immunity barrier has been transgressed, it manifests as possibly pyrexia (increased temperature, fever), throat pain, muscle pain, lethargy, etc. Once the coronavirus enters the respiratory system cells, one will start feeling breathless and hypoxic due to the body's inflammatory response, and a resultant impending cytokine storm can ensue. This is the cause for fatality.

Covid has affected all of us, but none more than the lower middle class and the marginalized. They, especially, should know that the inexpensive but definite answers are right in their kitchen. No chemical drug exists that can do what turmeric, ginger, garlic and lemon are capable of. Anybody who is shunning the above is because he or she has not used it.

If all of the above are not available, then turmeric powder in water alone will avert the cytokine storm. Every hospital and ICU should be resorting to this, and amazing results will follow.

Handling of Pyrexia

In Covid infection, fever is of moderate grade. It is a misjudgment to treat the fever. Rise in temperature enhances the immune system and lowers viral replication and bacterial growth. Therefore, one should not be in a hurry to treat the fever. It is our body's own defence mechanism. As Hippocrates has said, 'Give me a fever and I can cure any disease'. Paracetamol and aspirin acidify the body and bring down immunity. There are many studies that show viral infections are prolonged when antipyretics (substance to reduce fever) are overused.

Anti-pyrexial drugs and unnecessary antibiotics acidify body cells and are immune-lowering to the body. Prescribing these is one of the common errors of modern times and is the tipping point towards a cytokine storm syndrome.

Yoga, Alkalinity and Immunity

Yoga is a 5,000-year-old Indian tradition, being practised in some form in every country on earth now. It is more than a physical exercise. It unites the body and mind. It teaches one to breathe correctly and to make use of one's lung capacity maximally.

A practising yogi would be in an alkaline state. Anyone practising yoga goes into an alkaline, non-inflammatory state and easily goes up the alkaline ladder.

Yoga suppresses all inflammatory pathways and is the answer for preventing and curing lifestyle diseases.

It is impossible for anyone practising 10 *asanas* daily or doing surya namaskar daily to go into a cytokine storm syndrome which we are seeing

Beating the Cytokine Storm in Covid

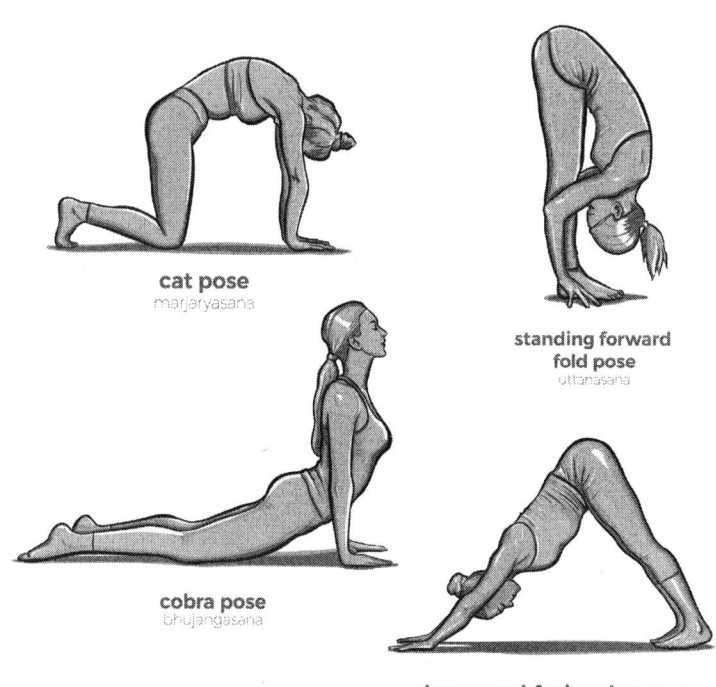

Designed by natalka_dmitrova/Freepik

now. Individuals who know yoga should be regularly practising it for 30 minutes daily in these times. For non-starters this is the time to start. Learn the basic breathing technique, '*Om*' chant, and start doing the *padhasana, sarvaangasana, matsyasana*, cobra pose, dog pose and *surya namaskar*.

The time has come for yoga to be taught to all medical students and a certain level of practice and understanding of yoga to be made mandatory to pass MBBS (Bachelor of Medicine, Bachelor of Surgery). It is only then that the evolving doctor will understand yoga as a preventive, therapeutic and wellness tool.

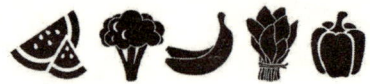

6

Alkaline Superfoods

*Woe to those who call evil good
and good evil, who put darkness
for light and light for darkness...*
Isaiah 5: 20

We have money, but have not organic food to eat: we travel on jets, but have not healthy air to breathe. We have solutions for all ailments from earth's own products but we fail to see. Such are the current times.

Our soil has been chemicalized with chemical fertilizers and pesticides. Therefore, the soil produce now does not have the same nutritional value it had a century ago. With cooking, heating and boiling we further reduce the nutritional content and are eating undernourished foods daily. Therefore, the last decade saw a lot of interest in consumption of raw organic foods. We have now moved forward to superfoods, and I believe in the next decade we will move further to superherbs.

Superfoods are nutrient dense foods. As the nutritional content of our day-to-day vegetables has been declining, we need to resort to superfoods, at least the smarter amongst us.

It is imperative that we understand superfoods and their role in maintaining our nutritional status, our alkalinity and immunity.

It is a lifesaving practice in current times to take superfoods and super herbs to alkalinize our body; for this, combined with a healthy lifestyle keeps our immunity in top shape.

Let me describe the best superfoods available to us currently.

Spirulina

Spirulina is a blue-green aquatic plant and is nature's complete source of nutrition. It was present on earth a billion years before life started on our planet. It was the initial source of oxygen for our atmosphere. The nutritional value of spirulina was known to our ancestors, but we are only rediscovering it again now.

The nutritional content of spirulina is shown below. No other single source of food can give this unique blend.

Being natural it is non-toxic and has been called the 'queen of all herbs'. Being water soluble, the absorption starts in the mouth and the protein is non-mucus forming and non-acid forming unlike animal and milk proteins. Its vitamin content is complete except Vitamin C.

It is the ultimate alkalinity booster, immune

Nutritional value of 1mg Spirulina

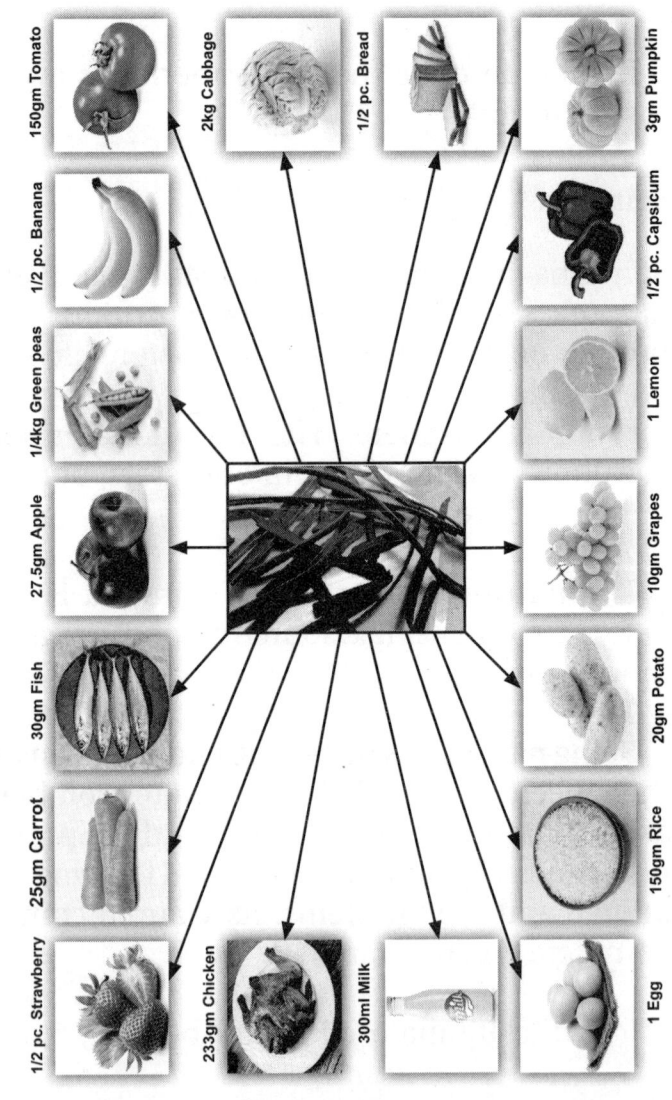

booster and body health booster.

Spirulina contains pure chlorophyll and phycocyanin (blue pigment protein). Chlorophyll, called the blood of plants, has the exact same structure as hemoglobin except that the core iron is replaced by magnesium. Chlorophyll is converted into hemoglobin easily in the body.

Phycocyanin gives spirulina the bluish tinge, and has a structure similar to bilirubin (a brownish yellow substance found in bile; it is produced when the liver breaks down old red blood cells). Like bilirubin, phycocyanin has free radical scavenging property and some researchers call this the wonder molecule.

Phycocyanin is hepatoprotective (prevents damage to the liver), neuro-protective (protects the nervous system from injury and damage) and has profound anti-inflammatory properties. These have been studied in detail and numerous papers are available. Phycocyanin helps combat the toxins in air from oil and gas, and toxins of heavy metals and nuclear isotopes.

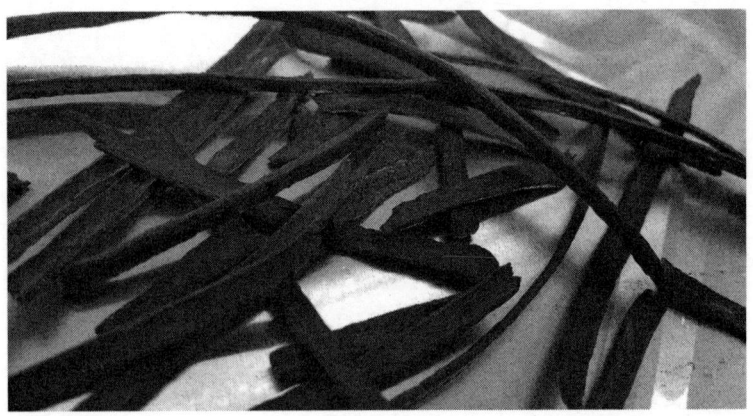

Image Courtesy: The European Space Agency

Spirulina is a *prebiotic*, promoting growth of friendly intestinal bacteria, especially lactobacillus and bifidus. We now know that our gut health is the predominant indicator of our immunity status, mental status and overall body health. All chemical drugs, especially antibiotics, alter our intestinal flora, and spirulina and all alkaline superfoods help restore this.

Spirulina also enhances bone marrow activity and production of T-cells, the natural killer cells. This enables the body to get natural protection against viral and bacterial attacks.

Many companies produce spirulina, and it is made available in powder form, tablets or capsules. In my experience, DXN is a company that produces this in its purest and organic form with amazing results which I see daily.

I believe a person regularly consuming spirulina cannot succumb to Covid. I am quietly confident that not a single regular consumer of spirulina on the planet would have had the cytokine storm.

All Covid patients and all of us should consume spirulina daily. In a person with ensuing hypoxia and impending cytokine storm; five capsules (300 mg each) of spirulina and a glass of turmeric powder water will reverse the hypoxia and abort the cytokine storm. If only the world knew and had faith in nature.

Ganoderma – The King of Herbs

The Pharmacopoeia of the People's Republic of China, written in the first century BC, documents the miraculous properties of ganoderma which is a red woody mushroom that grows horizontally

Survive Covid: By Staying Alkaline

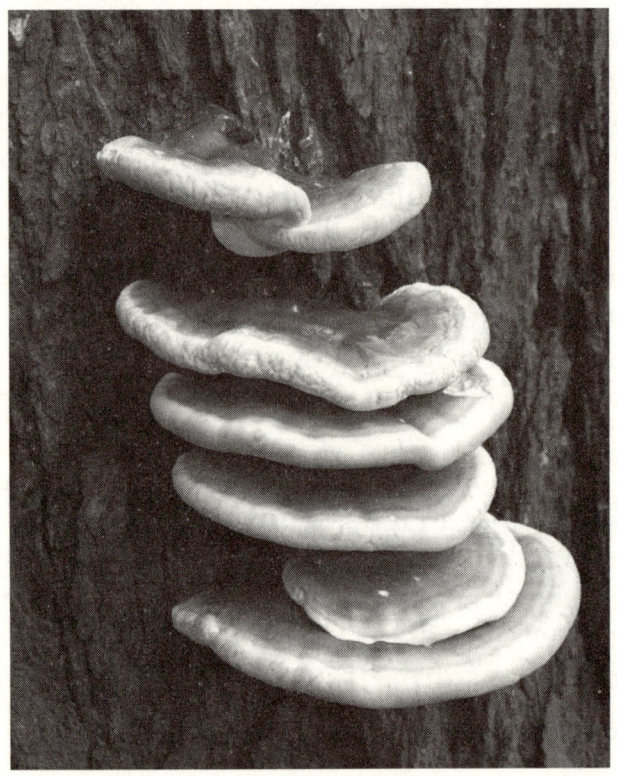

Reishi mushroom

on tree barks and is found in dense tropical rain forests with dim lighting and high humidity.

Ganoderma (also known as Reishi mushroom)

is the most alkaline of all foods on the planet. It upgrades body immunity, and with its adaptogen capacity normalizes every cell in our body. It is also called as the *herb of spiritual potency,* as well-being is followed by divinity and longevity. In human history there had been only few anecdotal reports but in the last few years numerous clear scientific reports and studies are emerging. More than 400 active ingredients and medicinal properties have been found in this mushroom. Adenosine, tripertinoids, ganoderic essence, organic germanium, polysaccharides are to name a few and the reader can refer to my previous book *Beyond Modern Medicine* or look up numerous emerging papers on this mushroom.

Adaptogenic effect is a term and property unknown to modern medicine. An adaptogen has the ability to enter every cell and correct any imbalances within.

We are living in a world of stress, environmental pollution, and consuming acidic toxic food replete with high sugar, cholesterol, salt, fat and chemicals daily.

Enormous resources are being spent all over the world in building hospitals and training doctors. It is wiser for all to be in a state of optimal health and make hospitals obsolete.

Ganoderma is produced by few organic companies and is available as powder form and as capsules. Many companies like DXN have blended ganoderma into coffee and tea, and these too help in profound health and immunity upgradation.

In our current ignorant acidic era of stress and lifestyle disease and with all of us walking around with low immunity status, we cannot afford not to be consuming this superfood.

Cordyceps mushroom, shiitake mushroom and lion's mane mushroom are also superfoods that boost the activity of white blood cells and help our immune system.

All the above superfoods are now available in the market and it is worthwhile finding them and consuming them regularly.

Alkaline Superfoods

Superfoods in our kitchen are coconut, moringa leaves, gooseberry, spinach leaves, which are all densely alkaline with dense nutrition and profound anti-inflammatory property than any chemical drug available.

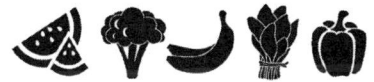

A Typical Alkaline Day

- Starting the day with cucumber juice and spirulina ensures an alkaline non-inflammatory beginning. One can have carrot juice or coconut milk on different days.

- It is equally important to keep toxic inflammatory food out of our diet. Breakfast should be around 8 a.m., lunch at 12 noon and dinner at 6.30 p.m. Early dinners are of prime importance.

- After yoga, it is always best to oxygenate the body with a walk or jog or a run.

- After the exercise, do calming yoga and meditation once again.

- It is a good habit to look at the early morning sun directly. The sun rays activate the retinal receptors and all the hormones for the day are released.

Happiness Quotient

- Keep the happiness quotient high throughout the day.
- Anger and negative thoughts bring in body inflammation. It is the time now to let go and forgive all.
- Many inflammatory bodies have some unforgiveness deep in them.

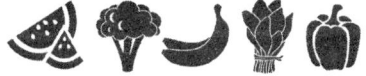

7

The Post-Covid Body Status

By the middle of 2021, every single human on earth would have had a Covid viral load. In alkaline immunocompetent individuals, Covid would not have transgressed the innate immunity and thus would have passed asymptomatically or as a simple passing cold and fever.

A small percentage would have had pulmonary symptoms, and many would have survived, especially if they had not resorted to antibiotics or steroids and overt usage of paracetamol. The survival rate would be highest among people who have resorted to alkaline food and lots of vitamins from fruits and Vitamin D activation from sunshine.

Amongst the post-Covid patients, almost all would have a period of lethargy and neuronal exhaustion. In some this would last a few days and for some these would be debilitating and continue for years and possibly lifelong if the root cause is not addressed.

The root cause of post-Covid syndromes is the leakage of inflammatory cells from the gastrointestinal tract. During the Covid response one would have inadvertently resorted to chemicals like paracetamol, non-steroidal analgesics and steroids and multiple antibiotics— all of which were never indicated in the first place. Gastrointestinal microflora is deranged in this situation and the inflammatory cells would leak into the main bloodstream. This usually lodges in joints of the body and causes joint inflammation. It can cause myocarditis (inflammation of the heart), myositis (inflammation of the muscles), and inflammation of any organ, hepatitis, pancreatitis, osteitis (inflammation of the bone), uveitis (inflammation of the eye), dermatitis, etc.—the timeline of post-Covid syndromes is only emerging.

The key here is to restore the gastrointestinal flora with alkaline diet and prebiotics, and not more chemicals for arthritis, which further compounds the leak. The increasing painkillers, steroids and antimitotic agents given to treat the joint pain will only worsen the situation and make it a lifelong condition, which results in the patient joining the arthritis industry of chemicals. At all stages, stopping the chemical drugs and going on earth's alkaline diet will normalize the situation.

During the post-Covid exhaustion, the body needs to regain the non-inflammatory alkaline status and this requires sleep. It is imperative that one sleeps double the normal sleep time. During sleep, the reparation of cells, rejuvenation of cells and removal of the inflammatory state occurs.

One should not resort to any form of exercise and not even yoga as the neuronal exhaustion is heavy and one would not be able to focus.

The key now is to resort to positive immune nutrition only and keep away from chemicals and all negative toxic inflammatory foods.

Vitamins C and D should be made available in plenty. Vitamin C—or ascorbic acid—is present in all fresh fruits. Having a freshly squeezed orange or lemon juice daily is worth a million drugs.

Vitamin D—the 'sunshine hormone'—is almost never nutritionally deficient but its activation requires sunshine. In other words, sun is the best source of Vitamin D. Hence spend at least 20 minutes in the sun daily. Vitamin D does not fit into the exact definition of a vitamin (vitamins are not produced in the body and we need to procure from food and does not need to undergo any process or pathway in the body). Vitamin D activation requires ultraviolet B (UVB) radiation and hence sunshine coming through glass windows would be devoid of this spectrum. One should stand in the open sun.

Depression, despair, feeling of insecurity, etc. follow the acidic inflammatory state of the body. The answer is to correct the inflammatory state with alkaline foods and superfoods and, as the inflammatory state changes the mind also becomes positive.

If not, as high as one billion people on earth could have post-Covid lethargic inflammatory states and would be treating the joint pains, muscle pains, lethargy, etc. with chemicals and never really will come out.

Vaccines are a Pandora's Box and each individual responds differently. Some post-vaccine individuals could also have lethargy and exhaustion as large numbers of Covid positive states are being seen now. The answer here again is to resort to rest and alkaline diet.

As the body comes out of the inflammatory acidic state to an alkaline non-inflammatory one, the mind also becomes calm and positive;

one starts the journey of going up the alkaline ladder. But if one resorts to chemical drugs, toxic processed food and negative nutrition, then it is really a one-way ticket on a dusty road and accelerated death.

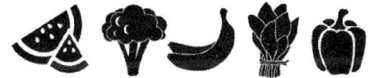

8

The Planetary Interconnection

*What you have learned is a mere handful;
What you haven't learned is the size of the world.
—Avvaiyar,[1] Tamil poetess, 3 Century BC*

Forty years ago, if anyone had written that zinc, manganese, chromium and other

---

[1] Avvaiyar was a Tamil poetess (Tamil Nadu is a southern state in India) who lived around the third century BC, or it could have been three poetesses who lived seven centuries apart—from the first BC to the seventh century BC. They lived in the times of great contemporary artists and poets the likes of who have not existed since. Her words stay true eternally.

trace elements are required for the body's vital functions, it would have been rejected as blabber and irrelevant information. Today we know the vital importance of these elements for the body's metabolism. Zinc, in particular, is vital for the immune pathways. In the near future, interest will move towards ultra-trace elements like silicon, gold, cobalt and germanium.

We are from the soil and go back to it. Our body needs products of the earth—all our essential requirements for health are made available to us from the soil by plants.

Organic germanium may be the next trace element that will create a lot of interest as an immune booster, an anti-cancer and anti-viral agent and much more.

Metallic germanium has its importance as a semiconductor in all transistors. Organic germanium is the non-metal form.

Ginseng, garlic, aloe vera, and Ganoderma lucidum—known as the Reishi mushroom—are medicinal herbs containing substantial amounts of germanium. This is possibly the main reason for their healing property. The amount of germanium in a plant varies according to the quality of the soil in which it grows. Adding germanium to the soil is known to enhance plant growth.

Germanium facilitates the movement of oxygen across cellular membranes to deliver oxygen to the cells. Dr Otto Warburg, the 1931 Nobel prize winner for physiology and medicine, discovered that cancer cells do not metabolize oxygen properly. He stated that cancer cells occur only in an acidic environment with a lack of oxygen. Organic germanium facilitates oxygenation of cells and this would retard the growth of cancer cells and even help return them to normal.

The therapeutic attributes of germanium include immuno-enhancement, oxygen enrichment, free radical scavenging, analgesia and heavy metal detoxification. It is postulated that 20 kilograms of organic germanium is enough to cure the whole world's cancer population.

The holy water of Lourdes, in the Sanctuary of Our Lady of Lourdes, France, is known to have miraculously cured thousands of pilgrims who visit the shrine. Chemical analysis of the water from the well there has shown that it contains unusually high amounts of germanium.

Germanium is known to regulate the electrical balance of the body. It is, therefore, called the balancer, especially by researchers of the mycelium (root) of the Reishi mushroom. Our body is youthful when all our cells are in communication with each other. We age as this intercellular communication diminishes. The electromagnetic radiation pools from mobile phones and Wi-Fi are interfering with our intercellular communications, and thus, prematurely ageing us. Herbs containing germanium are known to have profound anti-ageing effect. Organic germanium possibly allows plants to communicate with each other. The Reishi mushroom grows on trees that are dead or dying. Chinese and Indian traditional practitioners, 10,000 years ago, used to call the Reishi mushroom the 'King of all Herbs'. They also called it the 'Herb of Immortality' as an oxygenated alkaline cell keeps on living.

In future, there will be many attempts to produce organic germanium, but, as in the case of all vitamins and trace elements, it is the organic vegetable source that our body relishes and needs.

I have delineated organic germanium to get a window into the fact that all plants are in constant communication with each other electrochemically. All animals and birds communicate effectively with sounds and body language. As we evolve up the alkaline ladder we would enter into a state where we 'communicate' with plants and animals. Communicate may not be the appropriate word, it would be a state of awareness; we first have to let go of our human-centric state of thinking and realise our existence as part of all existence on the planet.

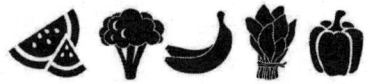

9

Earth Synchronicity, Earth Humility

Blessed are the meek, for they shall inherit the earth.[1]

—Mathew 5:3

There are many ongoing pandemics (other than the Covid-19) in our times, all interrelated and playing their own parts in lowering our

---

1. This possibly is the most discussed verse among the beatitudes. Meekness is humility towards earth, and all its inhabitants. Alkalinity brings this in everyone.

immunity—plastic pandemic, environmental pollution pandemic, chemical drugs pandemic, and ego pandemic, just to name a few.

Let me write about the ego pandemic. Ego is man-made—something that we inherited through life experiences. Acidic imbalance brings in a sense of false ego and pride—pride that we know everything.

I can urinate under a coconut tree and yet drink the most nutritious coconut water the next day. Can we manufacture anything like this? Of course, we can't; only Earth can. There is so much intelligence around us that we cannot even comprehend.

Admission of ignorance, along with respect and humility, to Nature is the need of the hour. Take some time out to observe Nature. You may end up learning a few valuable life lessons. Cheating nature is like poking a bear in the abdomen. We will end up paying a heavy price. The commonest nature-cheating events occurring now are:

1. Sleep

In current times of social media and WhatsApp etc, we stay awake late and carry our phones to bed and even toilets. It is scary when cities are named as 'a city that never sleeps'; one feels for the immunity of the inhabitants. Humans are diurnal and not nocturnal beings. As night approaches, melatonin, growth hormone and many other hormones are released and our body goes into a reparative and regenerative mode. At dawn with sunlight, skin receptors, retinal receptors, etc. awaken the body to start a fresh day.

When we lose our natural sleep, we are endangering our own health and immunity. From a point of view of maintaining adequate immunity, night is more important than day. Electricity has brought about remarkable changes in our lives, but we are paying an immunity price for having lost natural night.

2. Processed and Chemical Food

Organic food has now become a rarity. We have to be vigilant in our food sources. If not, we will be

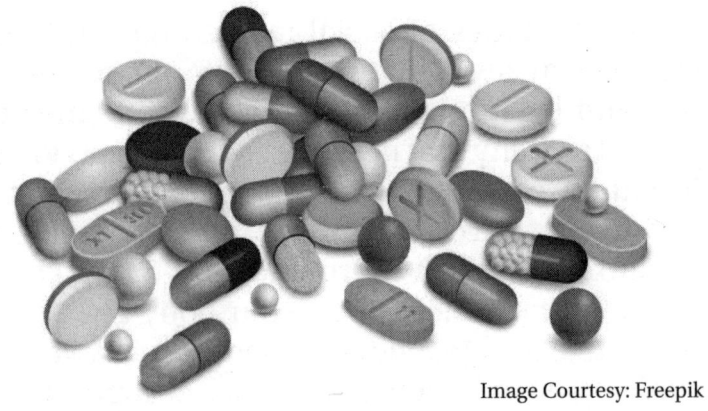

Image Courtesy: Freepik

eating to feed disease as opposed to feeding our cells. Processed food and snacks have high salt content, have zero or negative immune nutrition and contribute to body acidity, hypertension and atherosclerosis.

3. Chemical Drugs

All drugs make us acidic, with aspirin and paracetamol topping the list. They also alter the natural gastrointestinal microbial flora. The human body is wonderfully, fearfully and divinely created. We are cheating nature when we take chemical drugs. All drugs suppress symptoms temporarily, but the body pays a price in the long run. It is the physician's job to find out the root cause of the symptoms and rectify it, and not suppress the symptoms with drugs. We are in a digital world now, with all of us wanting instant results and immediate alleviation of symptoms; chemicals come in play here and we pay a heavy price for it.

We cannot cheat a fellow human being and get away with it, with even less chance when we cheat nature. We can never cheat nature and think of escaping responsibility.

Every world citizen has to unlearn a lot and be humble towards Mother Earth. We have to realize that to reach a state of top alkalinity and bliss, we have to offer ourselves to earth in everything we do. We have to keep nature robust and respect all her inhabitants.

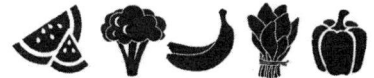

10

The Developed World and Alkalinity

When diet is wrong, medicine is of no use; and when diet is correct, medicine is of no need.

—Ancient Ayurvedic proverb

It is unfortunate that we use terms like 'developed' and 'developing' for parts of the world, based on the criteria of GDP, GNP etc. Nations with the least lifestyle diseases, where hospitals are not full, the prisons are not full, nations with more green grass than concrete filled cities, should be judged as leading nations of the world.

Nations that practice alkaline nutrition and an immune-friendly lifestyle will produce citizens with top immunity, and calm, responsible mindsets.

All leaders, therefore, should understand alkalinity, be alkaline themselves, and make this a priority in their own nations, and everything else will fall in line.

Royal Life

A kingly or a queenly life is a life without allergies, without daily productive coughs, without joint pains, with good bowel evacuation every morning, and with days filled with energy and positivity.

It is possible for every citizen to lead a royal life if they understand their alkaline diet and an earth-synchronous lifestyle.

A royal life is possible only with an alkaline/organic body and mind. We rightly opt for organic food; but are our own physical bodies kept organic? (If an educated lion was to eat me, would he consider me as an organic food or inorganic chemicalised toxic food?) Intake of any chemical makes our body acidic and inorganic. An alkaline diet and all vegetables have a detoxifying effect in extruding out the acidic toxins. This happens through urine, stool, sweat and lungs. Eating organic refers to not just the type of food, but it also refers to the timings of food and amount of food.

Mother Earth has given us everything around us to lead a disease-free royal alkaline life—it is just that we are failing to see it. If individuals and communities can understand the power of pH balance in an unbalanced world, then hospitals and prisons would become obsolete as alkaline bodies harbour calm, truthful and inclusive minds.

Currently, the world is talking about complying with non-pharmaceutical preventive measures

The Developed World and Alkalinity

like wearing face masks, maintaining physical distancing, practising hand hygiene and observing on-and-off lockdowns, apart from getting vaccinated and creating newer antiviral chemicals to kill the coronavirus (all these are unscientific methods and do not serve any purpose against an electron microscopical easily replicating virus). Unfortunately, there are neither talks about the benefits of connecting with Mother Earth and the benefits it brings about for our overall health nor a call to action for alkaline diet, alkaline tonic, or alkaline superfoods.

This era of ours will, therefore, go down in world history as a stupidity-filled, chemical-minded era where we forgot the power of natural immunity which is the only answer against all viruses and future pandemics. We Homo sapiens should understand that we need the Earth to survive, not the other way around.

Possible Scenarios Like Covid in Future

Fungi are another whole group just like viruses. They spread easily through spores and by fragmentation and budding. Our innate immunity keeps them at bay. If this innate immunity fails then the cellular immunity or T lymphocytes produce cytokines and neutralize the fungi spores and antigens.

The current Covid pandemic has provided us with an immunity map of the world, with more fatalities occurring in the developed world where lifestyle diseases are higher. Just as the viruses are ubiquitous so are the fungi. As the world's immunity deteriorates, fungi can emerge with various lesions. If B lymphocytes are in play against the virus (by producing antibodies), it would be the T lymphocytes that have to be in action against fungi.

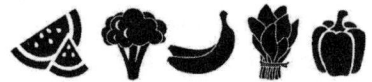

11

Will Humans Become Extinct? Quite Possibly

Are we on the verge of our own extinction? All signs suggest that we are. We have no one but our own recklessness to blame. Many experts believe that human extinction is only a matter of 'when' and not 'if'—thanks to overpopulation, environmental destruction, and climate change. If we continue disturbing the equilibrium between us and Nature, the next pandemic could perhaps ring the death knell for us!

Extinction of Dinosaurs 66 Million Years Ago

Historians say that dinosaurs roamed the earth from 230 million years ago till around 66 million years ago.

As originally propounded in 1980 by a team of scientists led by Luis Alvarez and his son Walter, it is now generally thought that the extinction of dinosaurs was caused by the impact of a huge asteroid or comet 66 million years ago, which devastated the global environment.

Other causal factors postulated are volcanic eruptions and the Deccan traps (one of the largest volcanic provinces in the world).

It is also postulated that dinosaurs were *on their way to gradual extinction,* before these catastrophic events occurred and these events were just the *tipping points.* We can never know for sure what caused the extinction of the dinosaurs.

- Did the dinosaurs ignore the basic laws of nature and become hyper predators? That is they not only preyed on herbivores but also on other predatory animals.

- Did they also have a gradual lowering of their immune status thus allowing viruses to cause inflammatory responses and ultimately causing their extinction?

- Did they also have an acidic ego pandemic?

- Are we now following the destiny of the dinosaurs?

No matter, however one thinks, raising an animal to kill (an animal that has its own brain, sensitivities and right to live), has to be morally wrong. Our toxic carnivorous mindsets have to change.

Plant proteins come with fibre, vitamins, antioxidants, that alkalinises the body and have a prebiotic effect that helps normalize our gastrointestinal microbial flora. Animal protein comes with zero fibre, no prebiotic effect, and acidifies the body.

If the asteroid impact was the tipping point for the dinosaurs, then the tipping point for this ongoing pandemic currently must be 4G and the upcoming 5G. Electromagnetic radiations are interfering with our body's intercellular electrochemical balances and communication, resulting in premature ageing and lowering of immunity. This could be the ongoing current tipping point.

The tipping point of any pandemic is formally thought to be (as we are witnessing with the Covid virus) when a virus strain mutates into a virulent strain and becomes more contagious. We all know that the cold flu strains at the beginning of the wet season are different from the strains at the end of the season.

Cold viruses are mutating all the time. It is their given property from nature.

Let us have a rethink. The influenza pandemic of 1918 had a mortality of close to 40 million people worldwide. It was a time when the world was devastated by the First World War which ended that year. The collective immunity of the world population, especially Europe, was down and this was the ***tipping point***. It is the lowering of immunity that made the virus appear demon-like and contagious.

Therefore, it is not a single person that starts a flu epidemic, rather, it is the collective lowering of immunity of the population that makes it a flu epidemic.

The world is talking of a second wave, third wave, etc. of Covid; demonizing the virus and projecting it as if it possesses Hitlerian plans and attacks. The high sugar intake has tipped the acidic balance and immunity of the Indian population, making it an ideal ground for the virus to attack again and again. It is important to take every step possible to keep our immunity ironclad.

HIV persons have their immunity lowered and are prone to getting pneumocystis carinii pneumonia infection (a serious infection caused by the fungus Pneumocystis jirovecii). This organism is a normal commensal in healthy individuals. If the HIV ward has numerous cases of pneumocystis carinii pneumonia, it would not be called an epidemic.

The same is happening now. The collective immunity of the world population has been gradually coming down, with the added impact of the electromagnetic pools we live in daily, topped with an acidic diet and immune-unfriendly lifestyle.

Exit Strategy for Covid-19

The only exit strategy has to be, *alkalization and upgradation of body immunity*.

It is a possible scenario in future that the world population could be coaxed into taking vaccines every six months for the varying variants of the coronavirus detected. It is mind boggling that the whole world is talking of vaccines and lockdowns and not about the simple ways to increase body immunity. Therefore, this problem is going to stay till we come to this realization.

Vaccines and masks are mandatory now. **I wish exercise, alkaline diet, and waking up before sunrise are also made mandatory for all.**

It may eventually come to survival of the alkaline, and extinction of the acidic.

POST NOTE

As this book is being written, the whole world is wearing masks. Masks were worn by immunosuppressed patients after kidney and liver transplants. Yes, we are doing the right thing, because now we are all immune suppressed of our own making.

There is not much point in identifying the new variants of viruses and in creating chemicals to kill these ubiquitous tiny viruses. These viruses are part of earth and our daily lives. The Earthly aroma that we perceive after a summer rain is from the soil bacteria. Seeds germinate once planted in soil because soil bacteria (rhizobacteria) provide them with the impetus through plant hormone-like substances from the soil. *There is only goodness around us and all our earth co-inhabitants are pure goodness. Evil is from within us; there is no evil around us or on earth.*

These viruses are tiny and capable of changing their own genome as they replicate, things we cannot do. We need to be friends with them.

For this, we have to upgrade ourselves, by upgrading our alkalinity and immunity.

12

The Way Forward

If I have not impressed on the reader that alkalinity, earth synchronicity and earth humility is the way forward, then I have failed in my book.

A few decades from now, chemical drugs would not have withstood the tests of truth and time and would become obsolete. This current time of ours will go down as a period when humans lost their way and will be a dark era in medical history.

Live each day with alkalinity and be earth synchronous.

An alkaline body and an alkaline mind will produce nations and continents that are disease free, conflict free, and with all inhabitants living in harmony. Nations would want their neighboring countries to do well and to do better than themselves—that is what alkalinity brings in. Preventive medicine is all that doctors would need to know. One could get upset with the physician if one develops hypertension or osteoporosis after seeing him for a few years as he should have known how to prevent it. Hospitals would not be needed. Let us start conquering each day of our lives with alkalinity and practice healthy living now.

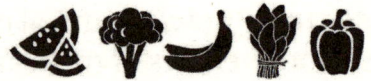

Conclusion

Let me conclude the whole matter. We cannot match the supreme intelligence of Mother Earth that surrounds us. We have to admit ignorance and submit ourselves to Earth and her magnificence.

Alkaline body, alkaline mind, alkaline societies, and an alkaline world is what we should all strive for. Alkalinity takes us deep into the very dawn of awareness, and we are able to connect with animals, plants and with everything around us. Life is then lived on a higher scale. An awareness full life is a life synchronous with earth and nature in every way. It is an all-inclusive life—one that is above truth and evil, above petty feelings of nationalities and religious constraints, above feelings of good and bad. It is an egoless, blissful state.

Every day is then bliss, as earth is what you want to be with, and earth gives you your daily bliss. As one sees nature's intelligence around us, one becomes humbled and ever grateful for this life opportunity. Mother Earth is our natural mother. Mother's love is the first and greatest gift for all living beings on the planet. From our first breath, to all our needs for health, immunity and longevity, are provided by Mother Earth. We have only to open our eyes.

Our body is from earth, given by earth. It is divine, and a holy sanctum. Would you desecrate the holy Bible or the holy Qur'an or the Shiva Linga? Our body should not be desecrated with man-made chemicals, for we will pay the price.

A world with all citizens in an alkaline balance is a disease-free, drug-free world with all living synchronously. Yes, this is very much possible in our lifetime.

I took the ride,
Looking for the answers,
Now I realize, I had known the answers,
Even before I took the ride.
Immunity cannot be had,
From chemicals, man-made.
It can fall, like a pack of cards,
Whilst natural immunity is everlasting.
The answers were looking me right in the eye
So, I had to write,
Mother Earth has all the answers,
Ignoring her, is at our peril.

Dr Eapen Koshy

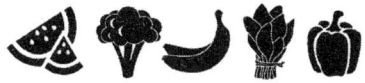

Common Questions

1. You talk about body pH and acidity. Is gastric acidity related to body acidity?

No. It is not.

Though gastric acidity symptoms are usually associated with individuals with acidic body, but it is not necessarily so. Gastric acid is as important as any of our innate immunity defence modalities. Gastric symptoms are due to an imbalance in the microbial flora and lowering of mucosal health and immunity. These have to be corrected with prebiotics and by upgrading body health. It is a pity that gastric acid production lowering agents are used world over by every doctor. One is actually lowering the innate immunity and welcoming more diseases. A combination of an acid production lowering chemical and a pain killer like paracetamol makes the body lose its first line of immunity. These can be the final tipping points in Covid patients in ICU.

2. Why are children and teens not affected, as of now, from the current Covid pandemic?

The tipping point of this pandemic, as I have

tried to explain, is the collective lowering of world immunity due to the environmental and dietary habits of the modern era. Obviously, kids and teens have not had enough time to get their immunity lowered. The greatest wonder of life is that we are all different. So are our individual immune responses. It is a Pandora's box.

3. Do you mean to say the whole world should embrace veganism?

If possible, Yes. Earth would then be heaven in the entire cosmos.

However, to live a disease-free healthy life it is advisable to have approximately 65 percent positive nutrition and 35 percent negative nutrition. If you wish to go to the top of the alkaline ladder, the nearer to 100 percent positive nutrition is a sure way to earthly bliss and spiritual potency. Try it: one life, one opportunity.

4. Lion is the undisputed king of the jungle. He is a self-proclaimed meat eater. What do you say to this?

It is an aberration, just as what happened to us. The most enduring camel gets its endurance from plant proteins only. Elephant, the biggest mammal, gets its energy and calcium from leaves, the horse does not ever have weak legs. The impala when chased by the cheetah can often outrun it with its zig-zag running. Elephants, horses, cows all have high volume bowel evacuations daily. Not a single lion or leopard has this pleasurable luxury.

As we are all interconnected, the day man changes his culinary habits, so will the lion. I am certain.

5. What is the role of drugs in our future?

Zero. No role.

All pharmacological drugs possess toxicity and only mask the symptoms. They therefore cannot stand the tests of time and truth. They will die out. And sooner, the better for mankind.

6. Will life change for ever or will we return to normal, like before the pandemic?

Life cannot return to normal unless we change our way of life and make drastic changes to the way we think. World immunity has reached a tipping point level, and more viruses and variants, and maybe fungi are bound to cause fatal inflammatory responses in the future. We have to respect Earth and all her inhabitants, show humility to Earth, for our own health and prosperity.

7. Will alkalinity cure all diseases?

The root cause of the disease has to be established and dealt with. It is often the dietary and environmental root causes that need to be identified. After rectifying this, alkalinity restores normality. An alkaline body cannot attract disease.

8. I tested positive for Covid thrice. What do I do?

I presume you did the RT-PCR test which is the gold standard now. Let me remind you that it does Not test your immune status or immune response. It does not establish whether you are symptomatic or even infectious. The genetic viral material from a past positive status may still be present.

It would be interesting to know if this test had been done on a hundred random individuals five years ago, how many would have been positive.

I advise you to relax, stay fit, stay alkaline, stay positive and get on with your life.

9. My nation's leader asked the entire country to ring bells and bang steel plates and vessels to drive corona away. Is there any basis for this?

Yes, there is. Alkalinity gives an immediate boost to our immune cells and also has immediate anti-inflammatory action. The immune system is closely associated with the neuronal and endocrine systems.

In prayer meetings, one sees wheelchair-bound pain-ridden patients suddenly getting up and walking without pain. It is due to the alkalinity induced by the pastors' words and the environment.

Having a glass of warm water with turmeric powder immediately brings in alkalinity and gives an immune boost. Similarly, sounds and vibrations bring in a calmness and immunity boost.

10. I have not understood your message of alkalinity. What do I do?

Do not worry. It only means you are not ready for it yet. I suggest you read again. I am sure you will be ready soon.

Reference List

'Difference between innate and adaptive immunity'. Microbiologyinfo.com

Adebamowo, Clement A, Donna Spiegelman, et al. 2006. 'Milk consumption and acne in adolescent girls'. *Dermatology Online Journal*, 12(4):1.

Alizadeh Fatemeh, Maryam Javadi, et al. 'Curcumin nanomicelle improves semen parameters, oxidative stress, inflammatory biomarkers, and reproductive hormones in infertile men: A randomized clinical trial'. *Phytother Res.* March 2018. 32(3):514-521. doi: 10.1002/ptr.5998. Epub 2017 Nov 28.

Amini, Paiman, Hana Saffar,et al. 'Curcumin Mitigates Radiation-induced Lung Pneumonitis and Fibrosis in Rats'. *International Journal of Molecular and Cellular Medicine.* 2018. 7(4): 212-219.

Asai, Kazuhiko. 1981. *Miracle Cure: Organic Germanium.* Japan: Japan Publications.

Cotton, R. and C. Milstein. 1973. 'Fusion of Two Immunoglobulin-Producing Myeloma Cells'. *Nature,* 244: 42-43.

Fenton, T.R., Eliasziw M. et al. 2008, 'Meta-analysis of the quantity of calcium excretion associated with the net acid excretion of the modern diet under the acid-ash hypothesis'. *The American Journal of Clinical Nutrition,* 88(4):1159-66.

Frassetto, L., R. Morris et al. 2001. 'Diet, evolution and aging—The Pathophysiologic Effects of the Post-Agricultural Inversion of the Potassium-to-Sodium and Base-to-Chloride Ratios in the Human Diet'. *European Journal of Nutrition*, 40(5): 200-213.

Janeway, Charles A. Paul Travers, et al. 2001. 'Principles of innate and adaptive immunity'. *Immunobiology: The Immune System in Health and Disease,* 5th edition.

Kohler, G. and C. Milstein. 1975. 'Continuous cultures of fused cells secreting antibody of predefined specificity'.' *Nature,* 256: 495-497.

Lardner, Anne. 2001. 'The effects of extracellular pH on immune function'. *Journal of Leukocyte Biology,* 69(4).

Leavy, Olive. 2016. 'The birth of Monoclonal Antibodies'.' *Nature Reviews Immunology*, 17(S1):S13-S13.

Leech, Joe. 2017. 'The Alkaline Diet: An Evidence-Based Review'. *Healthline.*

Liu, Ziteng and Ying Ying. 'The Inhibitory Effect of Curcumin on Virus-Induced Cytokine Storm and Its Potential Use in the Associated

Severe Pneumonia'. *Frontiers in Cell Development Biology*, 12 June 2020. https://doi.org/10.3389/fcell.2020.00479

Paul, Ketema N., Talib B. Saafir and Gianluca Tosini. 2009. 'The role of retinal photoreceptors in the regulation of circadian rhythms'. *Reviews in Endocrine and Metabolic Disorders*, 10(4): 271–278.

Rose Wellness. January 2021. 'Are you acidic or alkaline?' *Centre for Integrative Medicine.*

Schwalfenberg, Gerry K. 2012. 'The Alkaline Diet: Is there any evidence that an alkaline diet benefits health?' *Journal of Environmental and Public Health*, 2012: 630-727.

Soedamah-Muthu, Sabita S., Eric L. Ding, et al. 2011. 'Milk and dairy products production and incidence of cardiovascular diseases and all-cause mortality: Dose-response meta-analysis of prospective cohort studies'. *The American Journal of Clinical Nutrition.* 93 (1):158-71.

Sumner, Thomas. 2017. 'What killed the Dinosaurs?' *Science News for Students.*

Young, Robert O. and Galina Migalko. 2015. 'Alkalizing Nutritional Therapy in the Prevention and Reversal of any Cancerous Condition'. *International Journal of Complementary and Alternative Medicine, 2(1).*

What are the changes that you will bring about in your lifestyle for a healthy tomorrow?

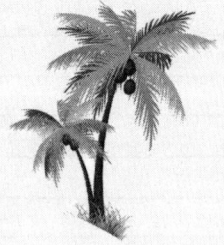 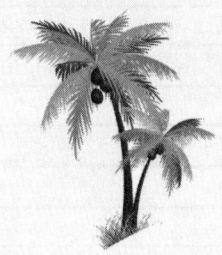

A Promise

There are 44 rivers in Kerala, a southern state in India. They originate in the Western Ghats, traverse the hilly terrains and empty into the Arabian Sea.

All proceeds from this book will go towards planting a billion coconut saplings along the banks of all 44 rivers of Kerala.